Alkaline Breakfast

The Ultimate Guide for Your Daily Healthy Alkaline Breakfast

Isaac Vinson

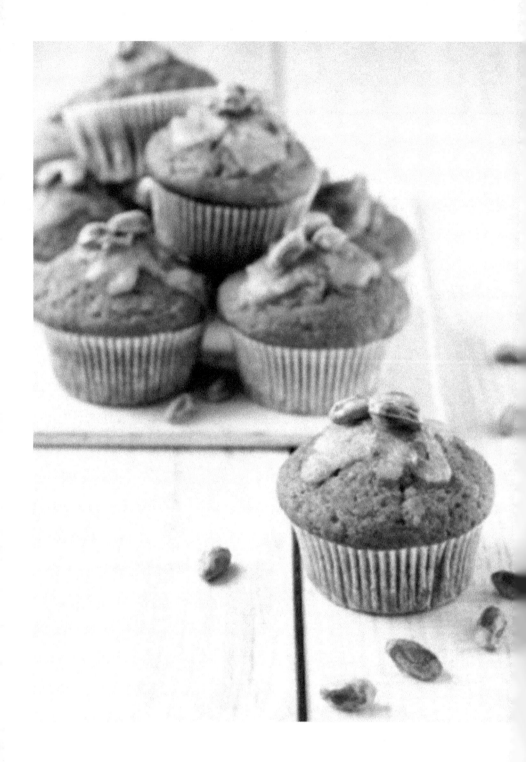

By reading this document, the reader agrees that under no circumstances is the author responsible for any losses, direct or indirect, which are incurred as a result of the use of information contained within this document, including, but not limited to, — errors, omissions, or inaccuracies.

Table of Contents

Layered Cabbage Roll Casserole

Preparation Time: 10 minutes
Cooking Time: 40 minutes
Servings: 4

Ingredients:
• 1 cup quinoa

• ½ red onion, finely chopped

• 4 garlic cloves, minced

• 4 white mushrooms, finely chopped

• 1 (28-ounce) can diced tomatoes, drained

• 2 cups low-sodium vegetable stock

• ¼ cup minced fresh basil

• 8 green cabbage leaves, whole

Directions:
1. Preheat the oven to 350F.

2. In a casserole dish, combine 2 tbsp. red onion, ¼ cup quinoa, 1 minced garlic clove, and 1 chopped mushroom. Add ¼ can of tomatoes, ½ cup stock, and 1 tbsp. basil. Stir to mix.

3. Top with 2 cabbage leaves. Repeat steps 2 and 3 until all of the

Ingredients are used up.

4. Cover and bake for 40 minutes.

5. Rest for 10 minutes and serve.

Nutrition:
Calories: 261

Fat: 2g

Carbohydrates: 51g

Protein: 12g

Mango, Quinoa, And Black Bean Casserole with Sauce

Preparation Time: 10 minutes
Cooking Time: 25 minutes
Servings: 4

Ingredients:
• 2 cups full-fat canned coconut milk

• 1 cup low-sodium vegetable stock

• 1 cup quinoa

• 2 cups black beans, drained and rinsed

• 1 mango, finely chopped

• ¼ cup minced fresh mint

• A pinch of sea salt, for seasoning

Directions:
1. Preheat the oven to 425F.

2. In a casserole dish, combine the stock, milk, and quinoa.

3. Cover and bake for 25 minutes.

4. Remove the dish from the oven. Mix in the beans, mango, and fresh mint.

5. Season with salt and serve.

Nutrition:
Calories: 573

Fat: 23g

Carbohydrates: 75g

Protein: 15g

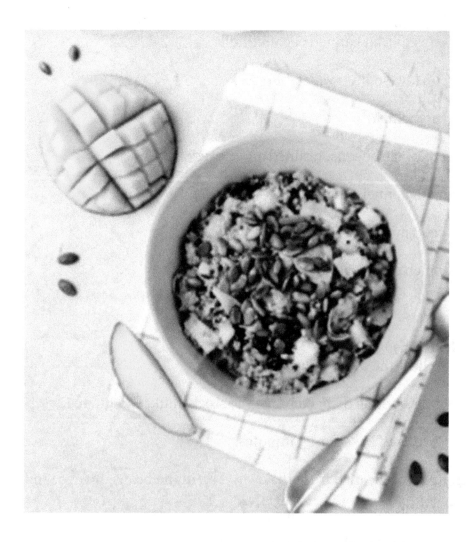

Pepper and Onion Masala

Preparation Time: 10 minutes
Cooking Time: 30 minutes
Servings: 2

Ingredients :
• 1 cup brown rice

• Boiling filtered water, for rinsing

• 2 tablespoons coconut oil

• 1 teaspoon cumin seeds

• ¼ teaspoon asafoetida

• ½ teaspoon ground turmeric

• 1 onion, rinsed and chopped

• 2 green chiles, rinsed and chopped

• 2 garlic cloves, chopped

• 1 (1-inch) piece fresh ginger, peeled and grated

• 3 tablespoons tomato paste

• 1 teaspoon chili powder

• Himalayan pink salt

• 1 bell pepper, any color, rinsed and chopped

• 2 tablespoons filtered water

Directions:

1. In a minor saucepan over average-low heat, associate the brown rice with enough boiling water to cover, and simmer for 25 to 30 minutes, until cooked. Drain and rinse with boiling filtered water.

2. Meanwhile, in a small non-stick skillet over medium heat, heat the coconut oil. Add the cumin seeds, asafoetida, and turmeric. Fry for 3 minutes, until golden.

3. Add the onion, green chiles, garlic, and ginger. Sauté for 5 minutes, until the onion is soft.

4. Stir in the tomato paste and chili powder, and season with salt. Mix well.

5. Add the bell pepper and water, and cook for 5 minutes.

6. Serve the rice with the hot masala.

Nutrition:
Calories: 520

Total fat: 8g

Total carbohydrates: 81g

Fiber: 6g

Basil and Olive Pizza

Preparation Time: 10 minutes
Cooking Time: 30 minutes
Servings: 4

Ingredients :
FOR THE PIZZA SAUCE

• 1 (15-ounce) can tomatoes

• 1 tablespoon extra-virgin olive oil

• ½ cup fresh basil leaves, rinsed

• 2 garlic cloves, chopped

• 1 teaspoon onion powder

• ¼ teaspoon dried oregano

• ¼ teaspoon dried sage

• ¼ teaspoon dried rosemary

• ¼ teaspoon red chili flakes (optional)

• 1 teaspoon Himalayan pink salt

• Pinch freshly ground black pepper

FOR THE PIZZAS

• 4 spelt flour pita breads

• 4 ounces vegan mozzarella, shredded

• 1 cup mixed veggies of your choice (tomatoes, eggplant, onion, green pepper, mushroom, etc.), rinsed and finely sliced

• 2/3 cup pitted olives, chopped

• 1 tablespoon extra-virgin olive oil

• 5 fresh basil leaves, rinsed and torn

Directions:
TO MAKE THE PIZZA SAUCE

1. In a blender, blend the tomatoes, olive oil, basil, garlic, onion powder, oregano, sage, rosemary, chili flakes, salt, and pepper on low until the basil and garlic are in very small pieces.

2. Transfer to a pot over middle heat and simmer for about 20 minutes, until the sauce reduces slightly and thickens.

TO MAKE THE PIZZAS

1. Preheat the oven to 500°F. Line a baking sheet with parchment paper and set aside.

2. Spread the pizza sauce evenly over the pitas. Top with the vegan mozzarella and scatter the sliced veggies and olives on top.

3. Bake for 8 minutes, or until golden on top.

4. Drizzle the pizzas with the olive oil and scatter the basil leaves over them. Freeze leftovers in an airtight container for up to three weeks.

Nutrition:
Calories: 400

Total fat: 10g

Total carbohydrates: 64g

Fiber: 5g

Sugar: 2g

Protein: 10g

Black Bean Chili

Preparation Time: 15 minutes
Cooking Time: 20 minutes
Servings: 4

Ingredients :
• 1 tablespoon coconut oil

• 1 small onion, rinsed and diced

• 6 mushrooms, cleaned and sliced

• 2 tablespoons ground coriander

• 2 tablespoons paprika

• 2 tablespoons ground cumin

• 1 tablespoon ground cinnamon

• 1 tablespoon ground nutmeg

• 1 tablespoon chili powder

• 1 (15-ounce) can tomatoes

• 1 can of black beans that is washed and exhausted

• 1 (15. 5-ounce) can kidney beans, rinsed and drained

• 5 cherry tomatoes, rinsed

• 2 tablespoons tomato purée

• 1 tablespoon raw honey or agave nectar

• ½ cup red wine or grape juice

- 3 squares dark chocolate, or 1 heaping tablespoon cocoa powder

- 7 ounces uncooked brown rice

- 4 tablespoons coconut yogurt, for serving (optional)

- 4 fresh cilantro sprigs, for serving (optional)

Directions:

1. In a great pan over average heat, heat the coconut oil. Include the onion and mushrooms, and sauté for 5 minutes. Stir in the coriander, paprika, cumin, cinnamon, nutmeg, and chili powder.

2. Add the canned tomatoes with their juices, black beans, kidney beans, cherry tomatoes, and tomato purée. Mixture to combine and carry to a simmer. Cook for 5 minutes.

3. Stir in the honey, wine, and chocolate. Turn the heat to little and simmer for 10 minutes.

4. While the chili cooks, cook the rice according to the package Directions. Rinse and drain.

5. Serve the chili above the rice, garnished with yogurt (if using) and cilantro (if using).

Nutrition:
Calories: 580g

Total fat: 5g

Total carbohydrates: 102g

Fiber: 18g

Sugar: 14g

Protein: 19g

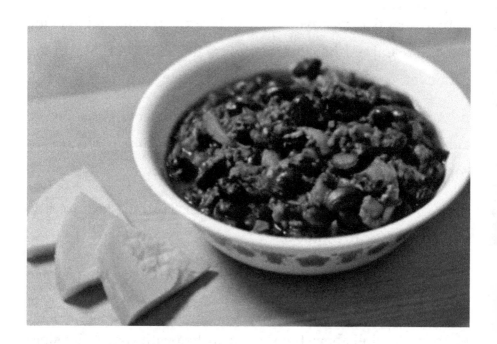

Mixed Lentils

Preparation Time: 15 minutes
Cooking Time: 30 minutes
Servings: 4

Ingredients :
• 2 tablespoons coconut oil

• 1 onion, rinsed and diced

• 2 carrots, rinsed and diced

• 2 celery stalks, rinsed and diced

• 1 sweet potato, rinsed and diced

• 1 cup dried red lentils

• 1 cup dried puy lentils

• 5 cups vegetable stock

• Himalayan pink salt

• Freshly ground black pepper

Directions:
1. In a large pot over medium heat, heat the coconut oil. Include the onion and fry for 3 minutes, or till softened.

2. Supplement the carrots, celery, and sweet potato, and cook for 2 minutes.

3. Add the red and Puy lentils and vegetable stock. Carry to a boil and lower the heat to simmer. Cook this for 25 minutes, or until the lentils are soft. Season with salt and pepper and serve.

Nutrition:
Calories: 330

Total fat: 10g

Total carbohydrates: 49g

Fiber: 20g

Sugar: 8g

Protein: 17g

Tomato Spelt Pasta

Preparation Time: 15 minutes
Cooking Time: 20 minutes
Servings: 4

Ingredients :
• 3 tablespoons extra-virgin olive oil

• 2 garlic cloves, crushed

• 1 onion, rinsed and diced

• 1 eggplant, rinsed and diced

• 2 zucchini, rinsed and diced

• 3 tomatoes, rinsed and diced

• 2/3 cup sun-dried tomatoes

• 2 teaspoons dried basil

• 1 teaspoon dried oregano

• 1 cup vegetable stock

• 1 tablespoon red wine vinegar

• Himalayan pink salt

• Freshly ground black pepper

• 7 ounces spelt pasta

• Boiling filtered water

Directions:

1. In a great pan over average heat, heat the olive oil. Add the garlic, onion, and eggplant, and sauté for 8 minutes.

2. Add the zucchini, tomatoes, sun-dried tomatoes, basil, and oregano. Cook for 8 minutes, stirring.

3. Stir in the vegetable stock and vinegar, and season with salt and pepper. Let simmer for a few minutes.

4. Meanwhile, in a separate, saucepan over medium heat, combine the pasta with enough boiling water to cover and cook for about, 10 minutes, until soft. Drain.

5. Serve the pasta with the sauce.

Nutrition:
Calories: 460

Total fat: 12g

Total carbohydrates: 75g

Fiber: 10g

Sugar: 11g

Protein: 17g

Green Tomatoes Crisps

Preparation Time: 14 minutes
Cooking Time: 16 minutes
Servings: 3

Ingredients :
• ¼ cup coconut flour

• Pinch of salt

• Pinch of pepper

• 4 green tomatoes

• 1 cup applesauce

• ½ cup almond flour

• ¼ cup olive oil

Directions:
1. First is to mix the coconut flour, salt, and pepper in a bowl. Mix the tomatoes. Toss until well coated.

2. In another bowl, pour applesauce. Add almond flour. Mix until well combined.

3. Heat the oil. Dip the tomatoes into the applesauce mixture and into the almond mixture. Fry tomatoes in batches until golden brown. Serve.

Nutrition:
Calories 113

Total Fat 4. 2 g

Saturated Fat 0.8 g

Cholesterol 0 mg

Sodium 861 mg

Total Carbs 22. 5 g

Fiber 6. 3 g

Sugar 2. 3 g

Protein 9. 2 g

Fruit Salad in Cider

Preparation Time: 11 minutes
Cooking Time: 16 minutes
Servings: 3

Ingredients :
• For the salad

• 1 piece, small apple, cubed

• 1 piece, small apricot, cubed

• ¼ piece, small grapefruit pulp, shredded into bite-sized pieces

• ¼ cup, loosely packed jicama, cubed

For cider sauce

• 2 Tbsp. apple cider vinegar, warmed in the microwave oven

• A dash of cinnamon powder

Directions:
1. Combine apple cider vinegar and cinnamon powder in a small bowl. Mix well.

2. Place salad **Ingredients** in large bowl; pour in cider sauce. Toss well to combine; spoon equal portions into plates. Serve immediately.

Nutrition:
Calories 123

Total Fat 14. 2 g

Saturated Fat 0.7 g

Cholesterol 0 mg

Sodium 661 mg

Total Carbs 22. 5 g

Fiber 6. 3 g

Sugar 2. 9 g

Protein 9. 2 g

Zucchini-Broccoli Stir-Fry

Preparation Time: 15 minutes
Cooking Time: 15 minutes
Servings: 4

Ingredients :
• 2 tablespoons coconut oil

• 2 tablespoons sesame oil

• 1 (2-inch) piece fresh ginger, peeled and finely chopped

• 4 garlic cloves, minced

• 2 onions, rinsed and chopped

• 1 head broccoli, rinsed and broken into florets

• 1 zucchini, rinsed and cut into long, fettuccine-like strips

• 3 scallions, white parts only, rinsed and chopped

• 1 tablespoon fresh basil leaves, rinsed and chopped

• 1 ounce coconut aminos

Directions:
1. In a wok or large skillet over medium heat, heat the coconut and sesame oils. Mix the ginger and garlic and sauté for 5 minutes, until fragrant.

2. Add the onion and broccoli, and cook for 3 minutes, until the onion softens slightly.

3. Add the zucchini, scallions, and basil. Stir to combine and heat for 4 minutes, until the vegetables are tender.

4. Remove the wok from the heat, sprinkle in the coconut aminos, and serve.

Nutrition:
Calories: 180

Total fat: 14g

Total carbohydrates: 13g

Fiber: 3g

Sugar: 4g

Protein: 3g

Pesto Soba Noodles

Preparation Time: 5 minutes
Cooking Time: 15 minutes
Servings: 2

Ingredients :
• 3 tablespoons extra-virgin olive oil

• 1 bunch fresh basil leaves, rinsed

• 1 bunch fresh parsley, rinsed

• 1 bunch fresh cilantro, rinsed

• 3½ ounces soba buckwheat noodles, cooked according to package Directions

• Himalayan pink salt

• Freshly ground black pepper

Directions:
1. In a blender, combine the olive oil, basil, parsley, and cilantro. Blend until smooth.

2. In a large bowl, combine the cooked noodles and sauce. Toss to coat, season with salt and pepper, and serve.

Nutrition:
Calories: 355

Total fat: 21g

Total carbohydrates: 36g

Fiber: 1g

Sugar: 0g

Protein: 9g

Quinoa Burrito Bowl

Preparation Time: 10 minutes
Cooking Time: 10 minutes
Servings: 4

Ingredients :
• 1 cup quinoa, rinsed well

• Boiling filtered water

• 1 can of black beans that is washed and exhausted

• 4 scallions, white parts only, rinsed and sliced

• 4 garlic cloves, minced

• 1 teaspoon ground cumin

• 1 teaspoon red pepper flakes

• Juice of 2 limes

• 2 avocados, peeled, pitted, and sliced

• Handful fresh cilantro, rinsed and chopped

 Directions:
1. In a small saucepan over medium heat, combine the quinoa with enough boiling water to shield and you then simmer for 8 to 10 minutes, until the water has absorbed. Drain, rinse, and set aside.

2. Meanwhile, in another small saucepan over low heat, stir together the black beans, scallions, garlic, cumin, red pepper flakes, and lime juice. Simmer for 10 minutes to warm.

3. In a large bowl, stir collected the quinoa and warmed beans. Top with the avocado and cilantro and serve.

Nutrition:
Calories: 420

Total fat: 9g

Carbohydrates: 70g

Fiber: 18g

Sugar: 2g

Protein: 10g

Banana Muffins

Preparation Time: 25 Minutes
Cooking Time: 20 minutes
Servings: 6

Ingredients

- ½ teaspoon salt

- 1 tablespoon vanilla extract

- 3 tablespoons ground flax seeds and 6-9 tablespoons water (egg substitute)

- 3 very ripe bananas, mashed

- ¼ cup oil

- 2 cups almond flour

- 1 tablespoon raw honey

- 1 teaspoon baking soda

Directions:

1. Preheat your oven to 350 degrees F, and mix the flaxseed, honey, banana, vanilla and oil.

2. In a different bowl, mix the baking soda, almond flour and salt.

3. Gently add the dry **Ingredients** into the banana mixture.

4. Spoon the batter into a greased muffin tin and bake for about 15 minutes. Insert a toothpick to check if it is done.

Nutrition:
Calories 140

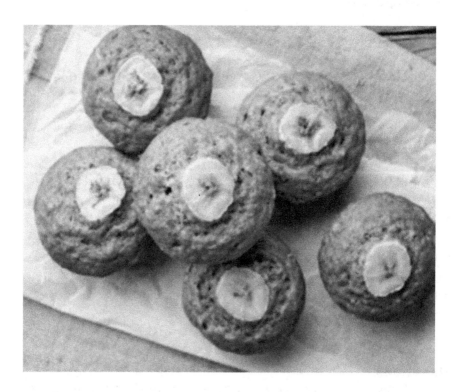

Flourless Banana Bread Muffins

Preparation Time: 20 Minutes
Cooking Time: 15 minutes
Servings: 9

Ingredients
- 3/4 cup almond flour/meal

- 2 tablespoons raw honey

- 1 teaspoon vanilla extract

- 1 tablespoon flaxseed plus 2 tablespoons water (combined)

- ½ cup rolled oats

- ½ teaspoon ground cinnamon

- 2 ripe medium bananas (200 g or a cup mashed)

- 2 tablespoons ground flaxseed

- ¼ cup almond butter

- ½ teaspoon baking soda

Directions:
1. Preheat your oven to 375 degrees F and spray 9 cavities of your muffin tin with cooking spray. Place aside.

2. Toss all **Ingredients** into your blender and run on high until the oats are broken down and the batter turns creamy and smooth.

3. Pour the batter into the muffin tins; fill them about 3/4 full.

4. Bake for about 10 to 12 minutes until the top of the muffins is set. Insert toothpick to check for doneness.

5. Let the muffins cool approximately for 10 minutes before you remove them. The muffins can keep in an airtight container for 10 days.

Nutrition:
Calories: 133

Super Seed Spelt Pancakes

Preparation Time: 15 Minutes
Cooking Time: 10 minutes
Servings: 3

Ingredients
- 42g flax seeds

- ½ teaspoon stevia extract

- 37. 5g sesame seeds

- ¼ teaspoon fine sea salt

- 80g chia seeds

- 164g buckwheat groats

- 1 ½ teaspoons ground cinnamon

- ½ teaspoon baking powder

- 30g pumpkin seeds

- 2 tablespoons almond milk

- 1 teaspoon coconut oil

- 1 teaspoon baking soda

Directions:
1. Grind the pumpkin seeds, sesame seeds, flax seeds, chia seeds and buckwheat groats into flour and keep ¼ of the seed flour for later use (not for this recipe).

2. Add 2 cups of the seed flour to a medium bowl.

3. Add in the rest of the Ingredients but not the coconut oil. Pour in more milk if needed to attain the right consistency.

4. Add coconut oil to a non-stick pan and place over heat.

5. Once heated, pour thin layers of the batter and flip once you see bubbles form on top.

6. Cook until all the batter is used up.

Nutrition:
Calories: 110

Scrambled Tofu

Preparation Time: 10 Minutes
Cooking Time: 15 minutes
Servings: 1

Ingredients
- 3 cloves

- 1 onion

- 1/2 teaspoon of turmeric

- Salt for taste

- 50g firm tofu

- 1/2 teaspoon of paprika

- 1 handful baby spinach

- 3 tomatoes

- 1/2 cup of yeast

- 1/2 teaspoon of cumin

Directions:
1. Mince the garlic and dice up the onion.

2. Toss the onions into a pan and let them cook over medium heat for about 7 minutes. Add in the garlic and cook for 1 minute.

3. Toss in the tofu and tomatoes and cook for 10 more minutes. Add in some water, cumin and paprika and stir well. Continue cooking.

4. When the dish is about to cook, add in spinach, stir and once wilted, turn off the heat and serve.

Nutrition:
Calories: 121

Ginger-Maple Yam Casserole

Preparation Time: 10 minutes
Cooking Time: 40 minutes
Servings: 4

Ingredients :
• 2 yams, peeled and cut into ½-inch chunks

• ¼ cup fresh ginger, peeled and grated

• 2 tbsp. avocado oil

• 2 tbsp. pure maple syrup

• 4 tsp. cardamom

• A pinch of sea salt

Directions:
1. Preheat the oven to 375F.

2. In a casserole dish, combine the yams, ginger, oil, maple syrup, cardamom, and salt. Mix well.

3. Cover and bake for 40 minutes.

4. Serve.

Nutrition:
Calories: 144

Fat: 7g

Carbohydrates: 20g

Protein: 1g

Ginger-Sesame Quinoa with Vegetables

Preparation Time: 10 minutes
Cooking Time: 30 minutes
Servings: 4

Ingredients :
• 1 cup quinoa

• 2 cups low-sodium vegetable stock

• 1 tbsp. tahini

• 4 tsp. fresh ginger, peeled and minced

• A pinch of sea salt, plus more for seasoning

• 2 carrots, finely chopped

• 1 red bell pepper, finely chopped

• 1 cup snow peas, stringed and halved

• 2 tsp. sesame seeds

• Sesame oil, for garnish

Directions:
1. Preheat the oven to 325F.

2. In a casserole dish, combine the stock, quinoa, tahini, ginger, and salt. Mix.

3. Add in the pepper, carrots, and snow peas. Mix well.

4. Cover and bake for 30 minutes.

5. Top with sesame seeds and a drizzle of sesame oil.

6. Adjust seasoning with salt and serve.

Nutrition:
Calories: 261

Fat: 3g

Carbohydrates: 46g

Protein: 10g

Vegetarian Pie

Preparation Time: 20 minutes
Cooking Time: 20 minutes
Servings: 8

Ingredients :
Ingredients for Topping

• 5 cups water

• 1¼ cups yellow cornmeal

• For Filing

• 1 tbsp. extra-virgin olive oil

• 1 large onion, chopped

• 1 medium red bell pepper, seeded and chopped

• 2 garlic cloves, minced

• 1 tsp. dried oregano, crushed

• 2 tsp. chili powder

• 2 cups fresh tomatoes, chopped

• 2½ cups Cooked pinto beans

• 2 cups boiled corn kernels

Directions:
1. Preheat the oven to 375 F. Lightly grease a shallow baking dish.

2. In a pan, add the water over medium-high heat and bring to a boil.

3. Slowly, add the cornmeal, stirring continuously.

4. Reduce the heat to low and Cooking covered for about 20 minutes, stirring occasionally.

5. Meanwhile, Prepare the filling. In a large skillet, heat the oil over medium heat and sauté the onion and bell pepper for about 3-4 minutes.

6. Add the garlic, oregano, and spices and sauté for about 1 minute

7. Add the remaining Ingredients and stir to combine.

8. Reduce the heat to low and simmer for about 10-15 minutes, stirring occasionally.

9. Remove from the heat.

10. Place half of the Cooked cornmeal into the Prepared baking dish evenly.

11. Place the filling mixture over the cornmeal evenly.

12. Place the remaining cornmeal over the filling mixture evenly.

13. Bake for 20 minutes or until the top becomes golden brown.

14. Remove the pie from the oven and set it aside for about 5 minutes before serving.

Nutrition:
Calories: 350

Fat: 3.9g

Carbohydrates: 58. 2g

Protein: 16. 8g

Red Thai Vegetable Curry

Preparation Time: 10 minutes
Cooking Time: 15 minutes
Servings: 4

Ingredients :
• 2 cups vegetable stock

• 1 sweet potato, rinsed and chopped

• 1 head broccoli, rinsed and chopped

• 1 eggplant, rinsed and chopped

• 1 zucchini, rinsed and chopped

• 1 red bell pepper, rinsed and chopped

• 1½ cups canned, full-fat coconut milk

• 1 tablespoon red Thai curry paste

• 2 kaffir lime leaves

• 1 (1-inch) piece fresh ginger, peeled and grated

• Himalayan pink salt

• Freshly ground black pepper

• 2 tablespoons coconut aminos

• Juice of 1 lime

Directions:

1. In a large pot over high heat, bring the vegetable stock to a boil. Add the sweet potato, broccoli, eggplant, zucchini, red bell pepper, coconut milk, curry paste, lime leaves, and ginger. Reduce the heat to low and cook for 10 minutes, stirring frequently.

2. Taste and season with salt and pepper. Simmer for 5 minutes more.

3. Remove the pot from the heat, stir in the coconut aminos and lime juice, and serve.

Nutrition:
Calories: 300

Total fat: 19g

Total carbohydrates: 23g

Fiber: 9g

Sugar: 11g

Protein: 7g

Thick Alkaline Minestrone

Preparation Time: 10 minutes
Cooking Time: 15 minutes
Servings: 2

Ingredients :
• 1 tablespoon coconut oil

• ¼ onion, rinsed and diced

• 2 garlic cloves, minced

• ½ cup sweet potato, scrubbed and cubed

• ½ cup zucchini, rinsed and cubed

• ½ cup eggplant, rinsed and cubed

• ½ cup carrot, rinsed and diced

• ½ cup canned beans, such as white, navy, or kidney beans, rinsed and drained

• 1 cup tomato juice

• ½ cup vegetable stock

• Handful fresh basil leaves, rinsed

• Himalayan pink salt

• Freshly ground black pepper

Directions:

1. In a large pot over medium-high heat, heat the coconut oil. Add the onion, garlic, sweet potato, zucchini, eggplant, and carrot. Sauté for 3 minutes.

2. Stir in the beans, tomato juice, and vegetable stock. Bring to a boil. Reduce the heat to simmer and cook for 10 minutes.

3. Stir in the basil, season with salt and pepper, and serve.

Nutrition:
Calories: 168

Total fat: 7g

Total carbohydrates: 25g

Fiber: 6g

Sugar: 11g

Protein: 4g

Sprouted Buckwheat Crepes

Preparation Time: 15 Minutes
Cooking Time: 10 minutes
Servings: 4

Ingredients
- 1 tablespoon pure 100% vanilla extract

- ¾ cup pure water

- 1 cup buckwheat groats- soaked overnight

- 1 tablespoon chia seeds

Directions:
1. Rinse buckwheat thoroughly and soak it in 1:2 parts water overnight.

2. Rinse then drain well the following morning.

3. Add all your Ingredients to a blender and process until smooth.

4. Add coconut oil to a nonstick pan over high medium heat and pour in a thin layer to the center of your pan. Swirl the pan to make sure the batter spreads out- the texture should be thick enough to hold the shape for flipping.

5. Once the top is not liquid, flip and cook the other side until browned.

6. Do this with the rest of the batter.

7. Serve with some sprouted nut butter, fresh lemon juice, hemp seeds or whatever you like.

Nutrition:
Calories: 202

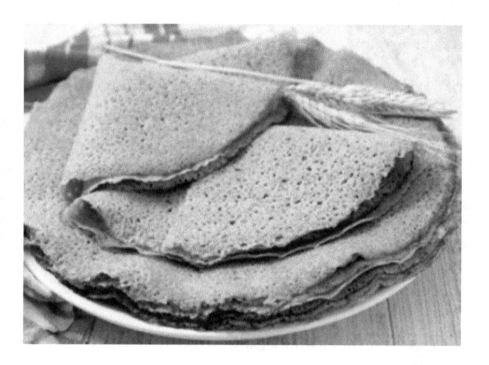

Butternut Squash, Apple Casserole with Drizzle

Preparation Time: 10 minutes
Cooking Time: 30 minutes
Servings: 4

Ingredients :
• 1 butternut squash, peeled, seeded, and cut into ½-inch chunks

• 2 Granny Smith apples, cored and cut into ½-inch chunks

• 1 white onion, cut into ½-inch chunks

• 4 garlic cloves, coarsely chopped

• ½ tbsp. avocado oil

• ½ tbsp. pure maple syrup

• 2 tsp. ground cinnamon

• ½ tsp. chili powder

• A pinch of sea salt

• A pinch of freshly ground black pepper

Directions:
1. Preheat the oven to 375F.

2. In a large casserole dish, combine the apples, squash, onion, garlic, oil, syrup, cinnamon, chili powder, salt, and pepper. Mix well.

3. Cover and bake for 30 minutes.

4. Serve.

Nutrition:
Calories: 123

Fat: 2g

Carbohydrates: 28g

Protein: 2g

Breakfast Salad

Preparation Time: 10 Minutes
Cooking Time: 15 minutes
Servings: 2

Ingredients
- 1/2 pack of firm tofu

- ½ a red onion

- 2 spelt tortillas

- 1 avocado

- 4 handfuls of baby spinach

- 1 handful of almonds

- 2 tomatoes

- 1 pink grapefruit

- 1/2 lemon

Directions:
1. Heat up the tortillas in an oven and once warm, bake for 8 to 10 minutes in the oven.

2. Chop up the onions, tomatoes and tofu and combine this. Put in the fridge and let it cool.

3. Now chop up the almonds, avocado and grapefruit. Mix everything well and place nicely around the bowl you had put in the fridge.

4. Squeeze a lemon on top all over the salad and enjoy!

Nutrition:
Calories: 80

Scrambled Tofu and Tomato

Preparation Time: 15 Minutes
Cooking Time: 15 minutes
Servings: 2

Ingredients
• 1 tablespoon coconut oil

• A little coriander/cilantro

• 285g regular firm tofu

• 2 big handfuls of baby spinach

• 1/2 brown onion (or red if you fancy)

• 1 handful of arugula/rocket

• Freshly ground black pepper

• 2 tomatoes

• Himalayan/Sea salt

• Pinch of turmeric

• A little basil

• ½ small red pepper

• A pinch of cayenne pepper

Directions:
1. Use your hands to scramble the tofu into a bowl then chop and fry the onion quickly in a pan. Dice the peppers and do the same thing.

2. Dice the tomatoes and throw them into the pan. Toss in a pinch of turmeric, and add the spinach. Add salt and grind in the pepper. Cook until the tofu is warm and cooked.

3. Throw in basil leaves, coriander, the rocket just when the meal is about to be done. Serve with a pinch of some hot cayenne pepper.

4. You can serve on some toasted sprouted bread and some baby spinach.

Nutrition:
Calories: 144

Spicy Jalapeno Popper Deviled Eggs

Preparation Time: 5 minutes
Cooking Time: 5 minutes
Servings: 4

Ingredients
• 4 large whole eggs, hardboiled

• 2 tablespoons Keto-Friendly mayonnaise

• ¼ cup cheddar cheese, grated

• 2 slices bacon, cooked and crumbled

• 1 jalapeno, sliced

Directions:
1. Cut eggs in half, remove the yolk and put them in bowl

2. Lay egg whites on a platter

3. Mix in remaining **Ingredients** and mash them with the egg yolks

4. Transfer yolk mix back to the egg whites

5. Serve and enjoy!

Nutrition:
Calories: 176

Fat: 14g

Carbohydrates: 0.7g

Protein: 10g

Lovely Porridge

Preparation Time: 15 minutes
Cooking Time: Nil
Servings: 2

Ingredients
- 2 tablespoons coconut flour

- 2 tablespoons vanilla protein powder

- 3 tablespoons Golden Flaxseed meal

- 1 and 1/2 cups almond milk, unsweetened

- Powdered erythritol

Directions:
1. Take a bowl and mix in flaxseed meal, protein powder, coconut flour and mix well

2. Add mix to the saucepan (placed over medium heat)

3. Add almond milk and stir, let the mixture thicken

4. Add your desired amount of sweetener and serve

5. Enjoy!

Nutrition:
Calories: 259

Fat: 13g

Carbohydrates: 5g

Protein: 16g

Salty Macadamia Chocolate Smoothie

Preparation Time: 5 minutes
Cooking Time: Nil
Servings: 1

Ingredients
- 2 tablespoons macadamia nuts, salted

- 1/3 cup chocolate whey protein powder, low carb

- 1 cup almond milk, unsweetened

Directions:
1. Add the listed **Ingredients** to your blender and blend until you have a smooth mixture

2. Chill and enjoy it!

Nutrition:
Calories: 165

Fat: 2g

Carbohydrates: 1g

Protein: 12g

Basil and Tomato Baked Eggs

Preparation Time: 10 minutes
Cooking Time: 15 minutes
Servings: 4

Ingredients
• 1 garlic clove, minced

• 1 cup canned tomatoes

• ¼ cup fresh basil leaves, roughly chopped

• 1/2 teaspoon chili powder

• 1 tablespoon olive oil

• 4 whole eggs

• Salt and pepper to taste

Directions:
1. Preheat your oven to 375 degrees F

2. Take a small baking dish and grease with olive oil

3. Add garlic, basil, tomatoes chili, olive oil into a dish and stir

4. Crackdown eggs into a dish, keeping space between the two

5. Sprinkle the whole dish with salt and pepper

6. Place in oven and cook for 12 minutes until eggs are set and tomatoes are bubbling

7. Serve with basil on top

8. Enjoy!

Nutrition:
Calories: 235

Fat: 16g

Carbohydrates: 7g

Protein: 14g

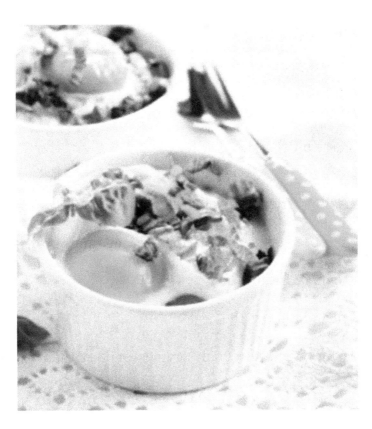

Cinnamon and Coconut Porridge

Preparation Time: 5 minutes
Cooking Time: 5 minutes
Servings: 4

Ingredients
• 2 cups of water

• 1 cup 36% heavy cream

• 1/2 cup unsweetened dried coconut, shredded

• 2 tablespoons flaxseed meal

• 1 tablespoon butter

• 1 and 1/2 teaspoon stevia

• 1 teaspoon cinnamon

• Salt to taste

• Toppings as blueberries

Directions:
1. Add the listed Ingredients to a small pot, mix well

2. Transfer pot to stove and place it over medium-low heat

3. Bring to mix to a slow boil

4. Stir well and remove the heat

5. Divide the mix into equal servings and let them sit for 10 minutes

6. Top with your desired toppings and enjoy!

Nutrition:
Calories: 171

Fat: 16g

Carbohydrates: 6g

Protein: 2g

An Omelet of Swiss Chard

Preparation Time: 5 minutes
Cooking Time: 5 minutes
Servings: 4

Ingredients
• 4 eggs, lightly beaten

• 4 cups Swiss chard, sliced

• 2 tablespoons butter

• 1/2 teaspoon garlic salt

• Fresh pepper

Directions:
1. Take a non-stick frying pan and place it over medium-low heat

2. Once the butter melts, add Swiss chard and stir cook for 2 minutes

3. Pour egg into the pan and gently stir them into Swiss chard

4. Season with garlic salt and pepper

5. Cook for 2 minutes

6. Serve and enjoy!

Nutrition:
Calories: 260

Fat: 21g

Carbohydrates: 4g

Protein: 14g

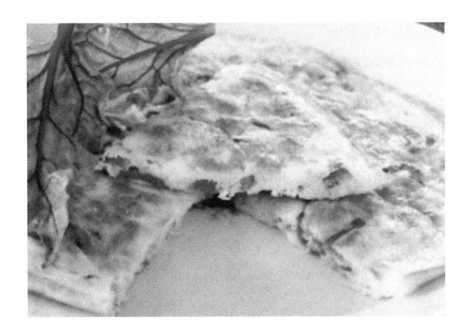

Cheesy Low-Carb Omelet

Preparation Time: 5 minutes
Cooking Time: 5 minutes
Servings: 5

Ingredients
- 2 whole eggs

- 1 tablespoon water

- 1 tablespoon butter

- 3 thin slices salami

- 5 fresh basil leaves

- 5 thin slices, fresh ripe tomatoes

- 2 ounces fresh mozzarella cheese

- Salt and pepper as needed

Directions:
1. Take a small bowl and whisk in eggs and water

2. Take a non-stick Sauté pan and place it over medium heat, add butter and let it melt

3. Pour egg mixture and cook for 30 seconds

4. Spread salami slices on half of egg mix and top with cheese, tomatoes, basil slices

5. Season with salt and pepper according to your taste

6. Cook for 2 minutes and fold the egg with the empty half

7. Cover and cook on LOW for 1 minute

8. Serve and enjoy!

Nutrition:
• Calories: 451

• Fat: 36g

• Carbohydrates: 3g

• Protein:33g

Yogurt and Kale Smoothie

Servings: 1
Preparation Time: 10 minutes

Ingredients :
• 1 cup whole milk yogurt

• 1 cup baby kale greens

• 1 pack stevia

• 1 tablespoon MCT oil

• 1 tablespoon sunflower seeds

• 1 cup of water

Directions:
1. Add listed Ingredients to the blender

2. Blend until you have a smooth and creamy texture

3. Serve chilled and enjoy!

Nutrition:
Calories: 329

Fat: 26g

Carbohydrates: 15g

Protein: 11g

Bacon and Chicken Garlic Wrap

Preparation Time: 15 minutes
Cooking Time: 10 minutes
Servings: 4

Ingredients
- 1 chicken fillet, cut into small cubes

- 8-9 thin slices bacon, cut to fit cubes

- 6 garlic cloves, minced

Directions:
1. Preheat your oven to 400 degrees F

2. Line a baking tray with aluminum foil

3. Add minced garlic to a bowl and rub each chicken piece with it

4. Wrap bacon piece around each garlic chicken bite

5. Secure with toothpick

6. Transfer bites to the baking sheet, keeping a little bit of space between them

7. Bake for about 15-20 minutes until crispy

8. Serve and enjoy!

Nutrition:
• Calories: 260

• Fat: 19g

• Carbohydrates: 5g

• Protein: 22g

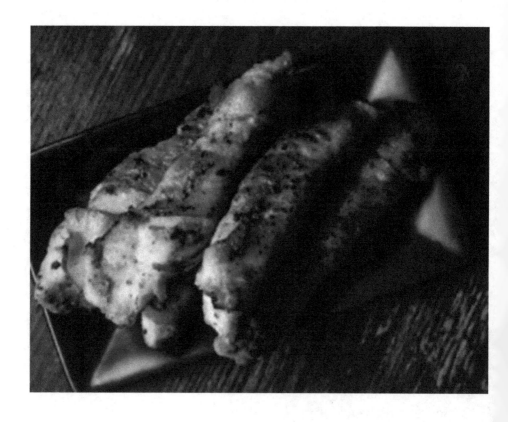

Grilled Chicken Platter

Preparation Time: 5 minutes
Cooking Time: 10 minutes
Servings: 6

Ingredients

• 3 large chicken breast, sliced half lengthwise

• 10-ounce spinach, frozen and drained

• 3-ounce mozzarella cheese, part-skim

• 1/2 a cup of roasted red peppers, cut in long strips

• 1 teaspoon of olive oil

• 2 garlic cloves, minced

• Salt and pepper as needed

Directions:

1. Preheat your oven to 400 degrees Fahrenheit

2. Slice 3 chicken breast lengthwise

3. Take a non-stick pan and grease with cooking spray

4. Bake for 2-3 minutes each side

5. Take another skillet and cook spinach and garlic in oil for 3 minutes

6. Place chicken on an oven pan and top with spinach, roasted peppers, and mozzarella

7. Bake until the cheese melted

8. Enjoy!

Nutrition:
Calories: 195

Fat: 7g

Net Carbohydrates: 3g

Protein: 30g

Parsley Chicken Breast

Preparation Time: 10 minutes
Cooking Time: 40 minutes
Servings: 4

Ingredients
• 1 tablespoon dry parsley

• 1 tablespoon dry basil

• 4 chicken breast halves, boneless and skinless

• 1/2 teaspoon salt

• 1/2 teaspoon red pepper flakes, crushed

• 2 tomatoes, sliced

Directions:
1. Preheat your oven to 350 degrees F

2. Take a 9x13 inch baking dish and grease it up with cooking spray

3. Sprinkle 1 tablespoon of parsley, 1 teaspoon of basil and spread the mixture over your baking dish

4. Arrange the chicken breast halves over the dish and sprinkle garlic slices on top

5. Take a small bowl and add 1 teaspoon parsley, 1 teaspoon of basil, salt, basil, red pepper and mix well. Pour the mixture over the chicken breast

6. Top with tomato slices and cover, bake for 25 minutes

7. Remove the cover and bake for 15 minutes more

8. Serve and enjoy!

Nutrition:
Calories: 150

Fat: 4g

Carbohydrates: 4g

Protein: 25g

Mustard Chicken

Preparation Time: 10 minutes
Cooking Time: 40 minutes
Servings: 4

Ingredients
• 4 chicken breasts

• 1/2 cup chicken broth

• 3-4 tablespoons mustard

• 3 tablespoons olive oil

• 1 teaspoon paprika

• 1 teaspoon chili powder

• 1 teaspoon garlic powder

Directions:
1. Take a small bowl and mix mustard, olive oil, paprika, chicken broth, garlic powder, chicken broth, and chili

2. Add chicken breast and marinate for 30 minutes

3. Take a lined baking sheet and arrange the chicken

4. Bake for 35 minutes at 375 degrees Fahrenheit

5. Serve and enjoy!

Nutrition:
Calories: 531

Fat: 23g

Carbohydrates: 10g

Protein: 64g

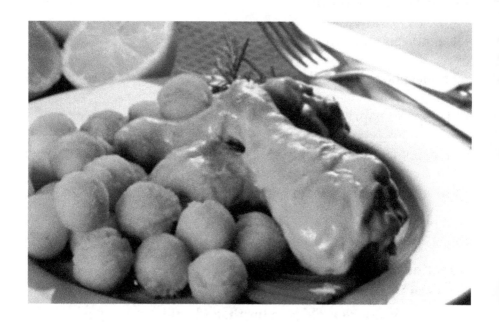

Balsamic Chicken

Preparation Time: 10 minutes
Cooking Time: 25 minutes
Servings: 6

Ingredients
• 6 chicken breast halves, skinless and boneless

• 1 teaspoon garlic salt

• Ground black pepper

• 2 tablespoons olive oil

• 1 onion, thinly sliced

• 14 and 1/2 ounces tomatoes, diced

• 1/2 cup balsamic vinegar

• 1 teaspoon dried basil

• 1 teaspoon dried oregano

• 1 teaspoon dried rosemary

• 1/2 teaspoon dried thyme

Directions:
1. Season both sides of your chicken breasts thoroughly with pepper and garlic salt

2. Take a skillet and place it over medium heat

3. Add some oil and cook your seasoned chicken for 3-4 minutes per side until the breasts are nicely browned

4. Add some onion and cook for another 3-4 minutes until the onions are browned

5. Pour the diced up tomatoes and balsamic vinegar over your chicken and season with some rosemary, basil, thyme, and rosemary

6. Simmer the chicken for about 15 minutes until they are no longer pink

7. Take an instant-read thermometer and check if the internal temperature gives a reading of 165 degrees Fahrenheit

8. If yes, then you are good to go!

Nutrition:
Calories: 196

Fat: 7g

Carbohydrates: 7g

Protein: 23g

Greek Chicken Breast

Preparation Time: 10 minutes
Cooking Time: 25 minutes
Servings: 4

Ingredients
• 4 chicken breast halves, skinless and boneless

• 1 cup extra virgin olive oil

• 1 lemon, juiced

• 2 teaspoons garlic, crushed

• 1 and 1/2 teaspoons black pepper

• 1/3 teaspoon paprika

Directions:
1. Cut 3 slits in the chicken breast

2. Take a small bowl and whisk in olive oil, salt, lemon juice, garlic, paprika, pepper and whisk for 30 seconds

3. Place chicken in a large bowl and pour marinade

4. Rub the marinade all over using your hand

5. Refrigerate overnight

6. Pre-heat grill to medium heat and oil the grate

7. Cook chicken in the grill until center is no longer pink

8. Serve and enjoy!

Nutrition:
Calories: 644

Fat: 57g

Carbohydrates: 2g

Protein: 27g

Chipotle Lettuce Chicken

Preparation Time: 10 minutes
Cooking Time: 25 minutes
Servings: 6

Ingredients
- 1 pound chicken breast, cut into strips

- Splash of olive oil

- 1 red onion, finely sliced

- 14 ounces tomatoes

- 1 teaspoon chipotle, chopped

- 1/2 teaspoon cumin

- Pinch of sugar

- Lettuce as needed

- Fresh coriander leaves

- Jalapeno chilies, sliced

- Fresh tomato slices for garnish

- Lime wedges

Directions:
1. Take a non-stick frying pan and place it over medium heat

2. Add oil and heat it up

3. Add chicken and cook until brown

4. Keep the chicken on the side

5. Add tomatoes, sugar, chipotle, cumin to the same pan and simmer for 25 minutes until you have a nice sauce

6. Add chicken into the sauce and cook for 5 minutes

7. Transfer the mix to another place

8. Use lettuce wraps to take a portion of the mixture and serve with a squeeze of lemon

9. Enjoy!

Nutrition:
Calories: 332

Fat: 15g

Carbohydrates: 13g

Protein: 34g

Stylish Chicken-Bacon Wrap

Preparation Time: 5 minutes
Cooking Time: 40 minutes
Servings: 3

Ingredients

- 8 ounces lean chicken breast

- 6 bacon slices

- 3 ounces shredded cheese

- 4 slices ham

• Directions:

1. Cut chicken breast into bite-sized portions

2. Transfer shredded cheese onto ham slices

3. Roll up chicken breast and ham slices in bacon slices

4. Take a skillet and place it over medium heat

5. Add olive oil and brown bacon for a while

6. Remove rolls and transfer to your oven

7. Bake for 40 minutes at 325 degrees F

8. Serve and enjoy!

Nutrition:
Calories: 275

Fat: 11g

Carbohydrates: 0.5g

Protein: 40g

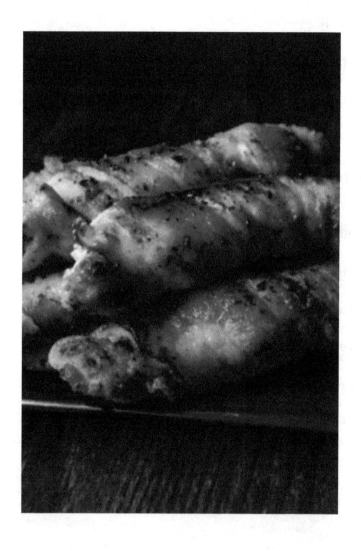

Healthy Cottage Cheese Pancakes

Preparation Time: 10 minutes
Cooking Time: 15
Servings: 1

Ingredients :
• 1/2 cup of Cottage cheese (low-fat)

• 1/3 cup (approx. 2 egg whites) Egg whites

• ¼ cup of Oats

• 1 teaspoon of Vanilla extract

• Olive oil cooking spray

• 1 tablespoon of Stevia (raw)

• Berries or sugar-free jam (optional)

Directions:
1. Begin by taking a food blender and adding in the egg whites and cottage cheese. Also add in the vanilla extract, a pinch of stevia, and oats. Palpitate until the consistency is well smooth.

2. Get a nonstick pan and oil it nicely with the cooking spray. Position the pan on low heat.

3. After it has been heated, scoop out half of the batter and pour it on the pan. Cook for about 21/2 minutes on each side.

4. Position the cooked pancakes on a serving plate and cover with sugar-free jam or berries.

Nutrition: Calories: 205 calories per serving Fat – **1.** 5 g, Protein – 24. 5 g, Carbohydrates – 19 g

Avocado Lemon Toast

Preparation Time: 10 minutes
Cooking Time: 13 minutes
Servings: 2

Ingredients :
• Whole-grain bread – 2 slices

• Fresh cilantro (chopped) – 2 tablespoons

• Lemon zest – ¼ teaspoon

• Fine sea salt – 1 pinch

Directions:
1. Begin by getting a medium-sized mixing bowl and adding in the avocado. Make use of a fork to crush it properly.

2. Then, add in the cilantro, lemon zest, lemon juice, sea salt, and cayenne pepper. Mix well until combined.

3. Toast the bread slices in a toaster until golden brown. It should take about 3 minutes.

4. Top the toasted bread slices with the avocado mixture and finalize by drizzling with chia seeds.

Nutrition:
• Calories: 72 calories per serving

• Protein – 3. 6 g

- Avocado – 1/2

- Fresh lemon juice – 1 teaspoon

- Cayenne pepper – 1 pinch

- Chia seeds – ¼ teaspoon

- Fat – 1. 2 g

- Carbohydrates – 11. 6 g

Healthy Baked Eggs

Preparation Time: 10 minutes
Cooking Time: 15 minutes
Servings: 6

Ingredients :
• Olive oil – 1 tablespoon

• Garlic – 2 cloves

• Eggs – 8 large

• Sea salt – 1/2 teaspoon

• Shredded mozzarella cheese (medium-fat) – 3 cups

• Olive oil spray

• Onion (chopped) – 1 medium

• Spinach leaves – 8 ounces

• Half-and-half – 1 cup

• Black pepper – 1 teaspoon

• Feta cheese – 1/2 cup

Directions:
1. Begin by heating the oven to 375F.

2. Get a glass baking dish and grease it with olive oil spray. Arrange aside.

3. Now take a nonstick pan and pour in the olive oil. Position the pan on allows heat and allows it heat.

4. Immediately you are done, toss in the garlic, spinach, and onion. Prepare for about 5 minutes. Arrange aside.

5. You can now Get a large mixing bowl and add in the half, eggs, pepper, and salt. Whisk thoroughly to combine.

6. Put in the feta cheese and chopped mozzarella cheese (reserve 1/2 cup of mozzarella cheese for later).

7. Put the egg mixture and prepared spinach to the prepared glass baking dish. Blend well to combine. Drizzle the reserved cheese over the top.

8. Bake the egg mix for about 40 minutes.

9. Extract the baking dish from the oven and allow it to stand for 10 minutes.

10. Dice and serve!

Nutrition:
Calories: 323 calories per serving

Fat – **22.** 3 g

Protein – **22.** 6 g

Carbohydrates – **7.** 9 g

Quick Low-Carb Oatmeal

Preparation Time: 10 minutes
Cooking Time: 15 minutes
Servings: 2

Ingredients :
• Almond flour – 1/2 cup

• Flax meal – 2 tablespoons

• Cinnamon (ground) – 1 teaspoon

• Almond milk (unsweetened) – 11/2 cups

• Salt – as per taste

• Chia seeds – 2 tablespoons

• Liquid stevia – 10 – 15 drops

• Vanilla extract – 1 teaspoon

Directions:
1. Begin by taking a large mixing bowl and adding in the coconut flour, almond flour, ground cinnamon, flax seed powder, and chia seeds. Mix properly to combine.

2. Position a stockpot on a low heat and add in the dry Ingredients. Also add in the liquid stevia, vanilla extract, and almond milk. Mix well to combine.

3. Prepare the flour and almond milk for about 4 minutes. Add salt if needed.

4. Move the oatmeal to a serving bowl and top with nuts, seeds, and pure and neat berries.

Nutrition:
Calories: calories per serving

Protein – 11. 7 g

Fat – 24. 3 g

Carbohydrates – 16. 7 g

Tofu and Vegetable Scramble

Preparation Time: 10 minutes
Cooking Time: 15 minutes
Servings: 2

Ingredients :
• Firm tofu (drained) – 16 ounces

• Sea salt – 1/2 teaspoon

• Garlic powder – 1 teaspoon

• Fresh coriander – for garnishing

• Red onion – 1/2 medium

• Cumin powder – 1 teaspoon

• Lemon juice – for topping

• Green bell pepper – 1 medium

• Garlic powder – 1 teaspoon

• Fresh coriander – for garnishing

• Red onion – 1/2 medium

• Cumin powder – 1 teaspoon

• Lemon juice – for topping

Directions:

1. Begin by preparing the Ingredients. For this, you are to extract the seeds of the tomato and green bell pepper. Shred the onion, bell pepper, and tomato into small cubes.

2. Get a small mixing bowl and position the fairly hard tofu inside it. Make use of your hands to break the fairly hard tofu. Arrange aside.

3. Get a nonstick pan and add in the onion, tomato, and bell pepper. Mix and cook for about 3 minutes.

4. Put the somewhat hard crumbled tofu to the pan and combine well.

5. Get a small bowl and put in the water, turmeric, garlic powder, cumin powder, and chili powder. Combine well and stream it over the tofu and vegetable mixture.

6. Allow the tofu and vegetable crumble cook with seasoning for 5 minutes. Continuously stir so that the pan is not holding the Ingredients.

Drizzle the tofu scramble with chili flakes and salt. Combine well.

7. Transfer the prepared scramble to a serving bowl and give it a proper spray of lemon juice.

8. Finalize by garnishing with pure and neat coriander. Serve while hot!

Nutrition:
Calories: 238 calories per serving

Carbohydrates – 16. 6 g

Fat – 11 g

Breakfast Smoothie Bowl with Fresh Berries

Preparation Time: 10 minutes
Cooking Time: 5 minutes
Servings: 2

Ingredients :
• Almond milk (unsweetened) – 1/2 cup

• Psyllium husk powder – 1/2 teaspoon

• Strawberries (chopped) – 2 ounces

• Coconut oil – 1 tablespoon

• Crushed ice – 3 cups

• Liquid stevia – 5 to 10 drops

• Pea protein powder – 1/3 cup

Directions:
1. Begin by taking a blender and adding in the mashed ice cubes. Allow them to rest for about 30 seconds.

2. Then put in the almond milk, shredded strawberries, pea protein powder, psyllium husk powder, coconut oil, and liquid stevia. Blend well until it turns into a smooth and creamy puree.

3. Vacant the prepared smoothie into 2 glasses.

4. Cover with coconut flakes and pure and neat strawberries.

Nutrition:
Calories: 166 calories per serving

Fat – 9. 2 g

Carbohydrates – 4. 1 g

Protein – 17. 6 g

Chia and Coconut Pudding

Preparation Time: 10 minutes
Cooking Time: 5 minutes
Servings: 2

Ingredients :
• Light coconut milk – 7 ounces

• Liquid stevia – 3 to 4 drops

• Kiwi – 1

• Chia seeds – ¼ cup

• Clementine – 1

• Shredded coconut (unsweetened)

Directions:
1. Begin by getting a mixing bowl and putting in the light coconut milk. Set in the liquid stevia to sweeten the milk. Combine well.

2. Put the chia seeds to the milk and whisk until well-combined. Arrange aside.

3. Scrape the clementine and carefully extract the skin from the wedges. Leave aside.

4. Also, scrape the kiwi and dice it into small pieces.

5. Get a glass vessel and gather the pudding. For this, position the fruits at the bottom of the jar; then put a dollop of chia pudding. Then spray the fruits and then put another layer of chia pudding.

6. Finalize by garnishing with the rest of the fruits and chopped coconut.

Nutrition:
Calories: 201 calories per serving

Protein – 5. 4 g

Fat – 10 g

Carbohydrates – 22. 8 g

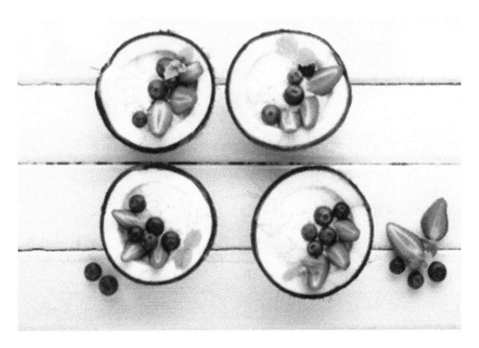

Tomato and Zucchini Sauté

Preparation Time: 10 minutes
Cooking Time: 40 minutes
Servings: 6

Ingredients :
• Vegetable oil – 1 tablespoon

• Tomatoes (chopped) – 2

• Green bell pepper (chopped) – 1

• Black pepper (freshly ground) – as per taste

• Onion (sliced) – 1

• Zucchini (peeled) – 2 pounds and cut into 1-inch-thick slices

• Salt – as per taste

• Uncooked white rice – ¼ cup

Directions:
1. Begin by getting a nonstick pan and putting it over low heat. Stream in the oil and allow it to heat through.

Put in the onions and sauté for about 3 minutes.

2. Then pour in the zucchini and green peppers. Mix well and spice with black pepper and salt.

3. Reduce the heat and cover the pan with a lid. Allow the veggies cook on low for 5 minutes.

4. While you're done, put in the water and rice. Place the lid back on and cook on low for 20 minutes.

Nutrition:
Calories: 94 calories per serving

Fat – 2. 8 g

Protein – 3. 2 g

Carbohydrates – 16. 1 g

Steamed Kale with Mediterranean Dressing

Preparation Time: 10 minutes
Cooking Time: 25 minutes
Servings: 6

Ingredients :
• Kale (chopped) – 12 cups

• Olive oil – 1 tablespoon

• Soy sauce – 1 teaspoon

• Pepper (freshly ground) – as per taste

• Lemon juice – 2 tablespoons

• Garlic (minced) – 1 tablespoon

• Salt – as per taste

Directions:
1. Get a gas steamer or an electric steamer and fill the bottom pan with water. If making use of a gas steamer, position it on high heat. Making use of an electric steamer, place it on the highest setting.

2. Immediately the water comes to a boil, put in the shredded kale and cover with a lid. Boil for about 8 minutes. The kale should be tender by now.

3. During the kale is boiling, take a big mixing bowl and put in the olive oil, lemon juice, soy sauce, garlic, pepper, and salt. Whisk well to mix.

4. Now toss in the steamed kale and carefully enclose into the dressing. Be assured the kale is well-coated.

5. Serve while it's hot!

Nutrition:
Calories: 91 calories per serving

Fat – 3. 5 g

Protein – 4. 6 g

Carbohydrates – 14. 5 g

Healthy Carrot Muffins

Preparation Time: 10 minutes
Cooking Time: 40 minutes
Servings: 8

Ingredients :
Dry Ingredients

• Tapioca starch – ¼ cup

• Baking soda – 1 teaspoon

• Cinnamon – 1 tablespoon

• Cloves – ¼ teaspoon

• Wet Ingredients

• Vanilla extract – 1 teaspoon

• Water – 11/2 cups

• Carrots (shredded) – 11/2 cups

• Almond flour – 1¾ cups

• Granulated sweetener of choice – 1/2 cup

• Baking powder – 1 teaspoon

• Nutmeg – 1 teaspoon

• Salt – 1 teaspoon

• Coconut oil – 1/3 cup

- Flax meal – 4 tablespoons

- Banana (mashed) – 1 medium

Directions:
1. Begin by heating the oven to 350F.

2. Get a muffin tray and position paper cups in all the moulds. Arrange aside.

3. Get a small glass bowl and put half a cup of water and flax meal. Allow this rest for about 5 minutes. Your flax egg is prepared.

4. Get a large mixing bowl and put in the almond flour, tapioca starch, granulated sugar, baking soda, baking powder, cinnamon, nutmeg, cloves, and salt. Mix well to combine.

5. Conform a well in the middle of the flour mixture and stream in the coconut oil, vanilla extract, and flax egg. Mix well to conform a mushy dough.

Then put in the chopped carrots and mashed banana. Mix until well-combined.

6. Make use of a spoon to scoop out an equal amount of mixture into 8 muffin cups.

7. Position the muffin tray in the oven and allow it to bake for about 40 minutes.

8. Extract the tray from the microwave and allow the muffins to stand for about 10 minutes.

9. Extract the muffin cups from the tray and allow them to chill until they reach room degree of hotness and coldness.

10. Serve and enjoy!

Nutrition:
Calories: 189 calories per serving

Fat – 13. 9 g

Protein – 3. 8 g

Carbohydrates – 17. 3 g

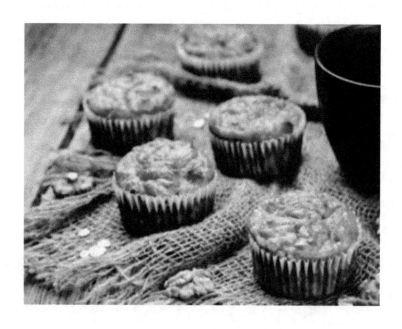

Vegetable Noodles Stir-Fry

Preparation Time: 10 minutes
Cooking Time: 40 minutes
Servings: 4

Ingredients :
• White sweet potato – 1 pound

• Zucchini – 8 ounces

• Garlic cloves (finely chopped) – 2 large

• Vegetable broth – 2 tablespoons

• Salt – as per taste

• Carrots – 8 ounces

• Shallot (finely chopped) – 1

• Red chili (finely chopped) – 1

• Olive oil – 1 tablespoon

• Pepper – as per taste

Directions:
1. Begin by scrapping the carrots and sweet potato. Make Use a spiralizer to make noodles out of the sweet potato and carrots.

2. Rinse the zucchini thoroughly and spiralize it as well.

3. Get a large skillet and position it on a high flame. Stream in the vegetable broth and allow it to come to a boil.

4. Toss in the spiralized sweet potato and carrots. Then put in the chili, garlic, and shallots. Stir everything using tongs and cook for some minutes.

5. Transfer the vegetable noodles into a serving platter and generously spice with pepper and salt.

6. Finalize by sprinkling olive oil over the noodles. Serve while hot!

Nutrition:
Calories: 169 calories per serving

Fat – 3. 7 g

Protein – 3. 6 g

Carbohydrates – 31. 2 g

Berry-Oat Breakfast Bars

Preparation Time: 10 minutes
Cooking Time: 25 minutes
Servings: 12

Ingredients :
• 2 cups fresh raspberries or blueberries

• 2 tablespoons sugar

• 2 tablespoons freshly squeezed lemon juice

• 1 tablespoon cornstarch

• 11/2 cups rolled oats

• 1/2 cup whole-wheat flour

• 1/2 cup walnuts

• ¼ cup chia seeds

• ¼ cup extra-virgin olive oil

• ¼ cup honey

• 1 large egg

Directions:
1. Preheat the oven to 350f.

2. In a small saucepan over medium heat, stir together the berries, sugar, lemon juice, and cornstarch. Bring to a simmer.

Reduce the heat and simmer for 2 to 3 minutes, until the mixture thickens.

3. In a food processor or high-speed blender, combine the oats, flour, walnuts, and chia seeds. Process until powdered. Add the olive oil, honey, and egg. Pulse a few more times, until well combined. Press half of the mixture into a 9-inch square baking dish.

4. Spread the berry filling over the oat mixture. Add the remaining oat mixture on top of the berries. Bake for 25 minutes, until browned.

5. Let cool completely, cut into 12 pieces, and serve. Store in a covered container for up to 5 days.

Nutrition:
calories: 201;
total fat: 10g;
saturated fat: 1g;
protein: 5g;
carbs: 26g;
sugar: 9g;
fiber: 5g;
cholesterol: 16mg;
sodium: 8mg

CPSIA information can be obtained
at www.ICGtesting.com
Printed in the USA
BVHW010951200521
R12259500001B/R122595PG607359BVX00025B/20